Weight Loss Motivation for Women

Change Your Mindset, Stop Torturing Yourself with Perfectionism, and Create Super Healthy Habits You Enjoy

by Elena Garcia

Copyright Elena Garcia © 2016

www.YourWellnessBooks.com

All rights reserved. No part of this publication may be reproduced, stored in a retrieval system, or transmitted, in any form or by any means, electronic, mechanical, photocopying, recording or otherwise, without the prior written permission of the author and the publishers.

The scanning, uploading, and distribution of this book via the Internet or via any other means without the permission of the author is illegal and punishable by law. Please purchase only authorized electronic editions, and do not participate in or encourage electronic piracy of copyrighted materials.

Your Wellness Books

Free Healthy Lifestyle Newsletter

Get new tips and recipes every week:

www.YourWellnessBooks.com

Disclaimer

A physician has not written the information in this book. It is advisable that you visit a qualified dietician so that you can obtain a highly personalized treatment for your case, especially if you want to lose weight effectively. This book is for <u>informational and educational purposes</u> only and is not intended for medical purposes. Please consult your physician before making any drastic changes to your diet.

Weight Loss Motivation for Women

[Life is a Balancing Act...7](#)

[Staying Motivated...17](#)

[Diet --- Ugh...21](#)

[Carving time for Cardio...42](#)

[Building Muscle...46](#)

[Exercising Your Soul...49](#)

[Sleep, Where Art Thou?...55](#)

[Final Words...58](#)

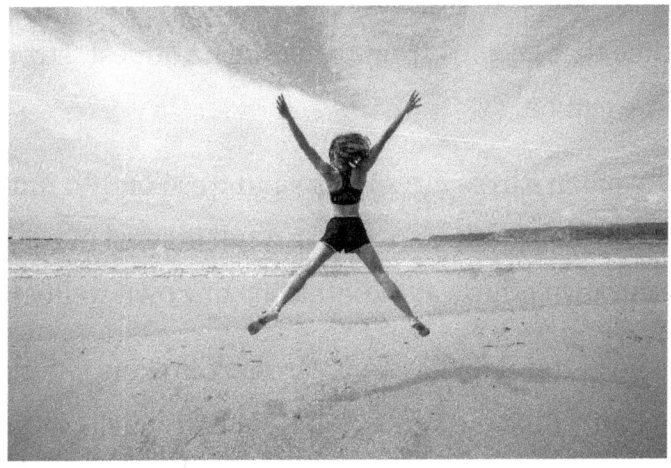

Life is a Balancing Act

Who wants to feel better and look better? What woman doesn't, right? I hear women **EVERYDAY** and **EVERYWHERE** saying, "as soon as I have more time", "as soon as the new year starts", "as soon as I have more money", "as soon as the kids are back in school", "as soon as I feel better... Then, I'm going to start dieting and exercising and taking better care of myself!"

Well, guess what? Those days we pretend are lingering out there in the future are not coming. Those are excuses we make all the time that keep us from being the healthiest, strongest women we can be.

Because women's lives are so busy and we spend so much of our time nurturing others, we have a full arsenal of excuses to combat our own efforts at maintaining our own wellbeing.

There is no better day than today to start making simple changes that will make you feel and look so much better. You've taken a first step by opening this book and admitting that your lifestyle could use some healthy changes!

Take one more important first step with me and reflect on where you are right now:

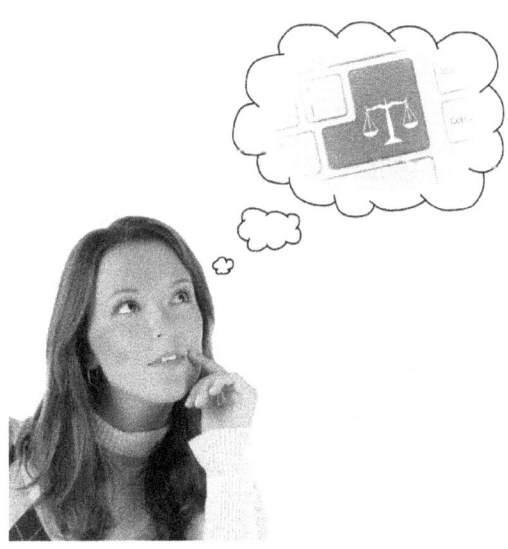

-Are you overweight?

-Do you need to lose just a few pounds, or do you need to shed 20 or more pounds in order to be healthy?

-Do you want to have more energy and feel better in general?

-Do you have a healthy diet but need more physical activity to become stronger?

-Are you in good shape but know you have some unhealthy habits that are holding you back?

-Do you need to find more quiet moments in your day for reflection and planning?

If you answered yes to any of these questions, keep reading! Just a few small changes in your day will reap huge dividends in the effort to become the best and healthiest version of yourself.

The most important thing is- be honest with yourself. In order to get where you want, you need to know where you are, right? You can be honest, realistic and positive. This is what this book is all about...

Women in general are perfectionist. We compare ourselves to what we believe to be the ideal woman, and when we fall short of that ideal, we beat ourselves up and we give up.

There is no perfect woman. She is a myth. I call it: deceptive marketing. They sell us this image to make us buy more and more products, ranging from beauty & fashion to weight loss pills, unrealistic cleanses, change your life in 7 days programs or be perfect in 3 easy steps. This is what clever marketers do. They create images of perfection that stay in our subconscious mind. Let's be real- there is no such thing as perfection.

Of course, I am not saying we should not strive for progress, we should. But first of all we need to overcome guilt-trips and chasing something that is not real.

Still want to believe there are perfect women? Point out those women you think are perfect, the ones you believe have it all, and I promise it doesn't take long to identify the flaws and burdens that they carry.

Stop comparing yourself to other women – the only woman you have to be better than is the one you were yesterday! Focus on where you are today and what your goals are for a more healthful lifestyle, a lifestyle that you deserve.

Reject everything that doesn't support you in your goals, including unrealistic expectations or deceptive marketing. You can be the best you can, just by switching off all those images of perfection and focusing on yourself; your self-love and intuition.

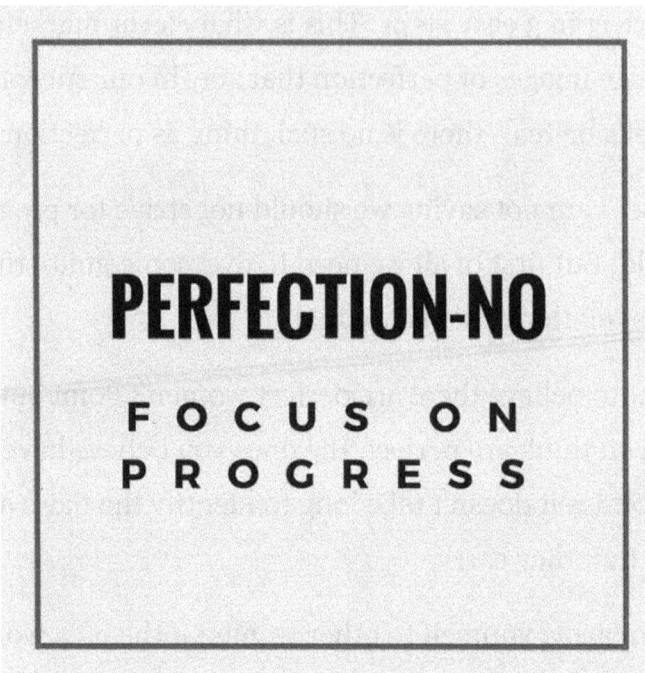

Another misconception we train ourselves with that stems from our perfectionism is believing we don't deserve the time it would take to become healthy.

Women are guilt mongers. We feel guilt over everything. How many times have you told yourself, "I'm not a good enough mother, wife, friend, employee, sister, ...?"

We stress out about everything we are not doing well enough ... except for taking care of ourselves.

We naturally feel guilty if we take time away from our other roles to focus on ourselves. It becomes a vicious circle because we don't feel strong and healthy, so we feel like we aren't performing any of our duties well.

The truth is you will be better at everything in your life if you carve out just a few minutes in your day to focus on your health. Don't be overwhelmed!

Start with small changes and as you grow stronger make more changes. I promise you will see results.

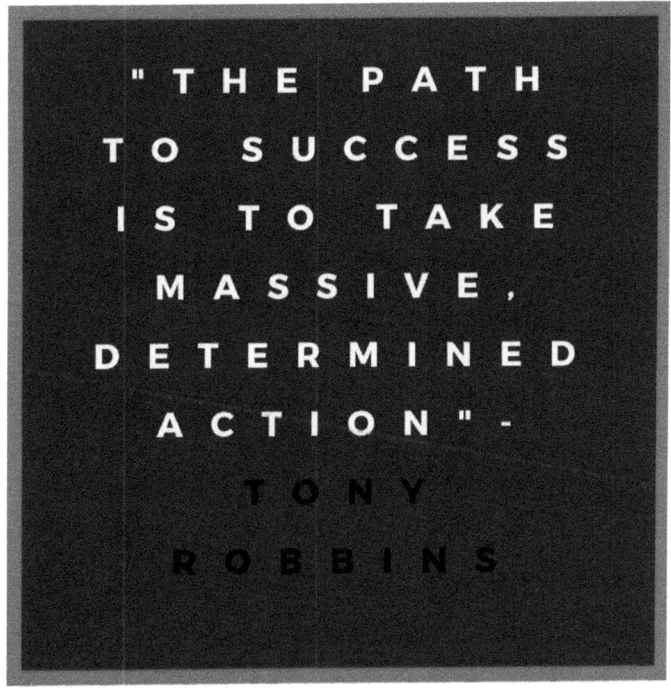

Life is hard and it doesn't cut any of us any slack! You deserve to be the strongest version of yourself so that you can juggle all that your life throws at you.

You deserve to feel good about yourself and enjoy the benefits of feeling strong and healthy. I talk to women who have achieved great weight loss to become healthy and those who only lost five or ten pounds to feel better, and they all have in common that they are incredibly proud of themselves!

It takes a commitment to put priority on our own wellbeing - to adopt practices to take care of ourselves and not just others. And, once we make that commitment, it is an accomplishment that has positive effects in every aspect of our lives.

Here's another important first step that won't cost you anything: think about your relationship with food.

What drives you when you make choices about what you put in your body? When do you eat and why?

Food should be a source of nourishment and we should eat for survival, but too often we use food as a reward or for comfort from the stress of our daily lives.

Many of us have developed an unhealthy relationship with food which has led to an unhealthy lifestyle.

We eat in an attempt to treat or alleviate a host of bad feelings we may be experiencing such as stress, loneliness, boredom, unhappiness, etc.

If this sounds familiar to you, start considering what motivates your diet choices and equip yourself to begin making healthy changes in what you eat and when you eat. This book is going to offer you some tools and options to get started.

We all know that the best life is one lived in balance and with moderation. Yes, you deserve a piece of cake at a birthday party or wedding.

Yes, you deserve a scone over coffee with a friend or a girls' night with cocktails. Those are all wonderful parts of living, but you should be able to enjoy them guilt free.

Occasionally treating yourself to something you really want is part of a balanced lifestyle.

If you treat yourself with poor choices every day, not only is it unbalanced but it will make you unhappy.

Making better choices daily allows us to enjoy those special times with fewer worries or anxiety. Being healthy is not about a prescribed diet, it's about learning to live a healthy lifestyle that allows you to enjoy the best version of yourself!

You deserve good health and the chance to enjoy the pride that comes from watching yourself transform into a stronger, healthier woman.

It takes planning and work, but it's guaranteed you will love the rewards. I want to challenge you to take the tools and suggestions in this book and begin making some changes that will lead to a better you.

If your goal is a major transformation, it'll take a lot of work, but you'll be so proud of yourself for making the effort.

Are you ready to start feeling like the best version of yourself? Let's get started – what do you have to lose?

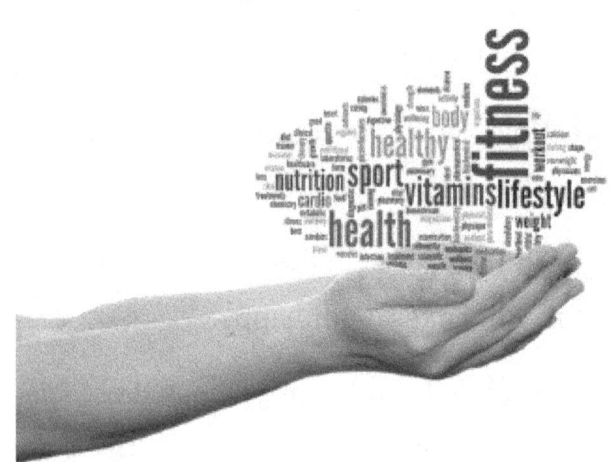

Staying Motivated

Let's talk about motivation for a bit – you'll enjoy this journey more if you plan sources of motivation along the way. Some changes are going to occur right away, but some will come more gradually.

Some of us are more impatient than others, and when we become frustrated with our efforts not producing desirable results, we give up.

Research tells us that once we start making healthier choices, we notice the effects in about two weeks. Those close to us notice in about four weeks, but people who don't see us daily won't notice for about six weeks.

So, we need a plan for staying motivated when we aren't experiencing the euphoria of success. Here are a few suggestions to get started.

1. Always keep in mind what motivated you to begin your journey finding a better you. Many mothers will say they want to have the energy to play with their children. Some of us want the energy to do our job better or be a better partner for our significant other. And, let's face it: vanity is a great motivator. Some of us just want to look better. We want to feel attractive. Whenever you feel like sliding back into your comfortable bad habits, think about what first made you step up and take on the

challenge to be better. You might not have reached your goal yet, but you are improving and getting stronger every day. Change won't happen back there in the Comfort Zone.

2. Surround yourself with people and things that support your journey. Connect with friends and family who have similar goals and build a support system. Share recipes and exercise plans. A workout partner is a great help, even if you just take a walk together a few days a week. There are hundreds of inspirational bloggers to follow who offer motivation, recipes, and lifestyle advice. Find a few that you enjoy and interact with their blogs. You'll learn so much and the different choices you find will keep you from getting bored.

3. Use technology! Fitbits are fabulous devices to get started. You can connect with friends and engage in healthy competitions – compete to see who makes those 10,000 steps most often. It'll also track your sleeping patterns so that you can at least become aware of how much rest you are getting. There are also hundreds of apps to choose from to help you with every aspect of a healthy lifestyle. My Fitness Pal and Map My Fitness remain top-rated, but a search will render hundreds of excellent options, many for free! You can

find apps that will help with recipes, music for your workout, meditation tips, or even a prescribed workout. If you are stuck indoors, go to YouTube for an abundance of workout video choices for any exercise and any skill level.

4. Preparation is also a great motivator. If you prepare for the journey, you'll be much more successful and you'll enjoy the trip a lot more. Take a few minutes at the beginning of each week and make a menu. Stock your kitchen with healthy foods and lots of choices so you don't get bored. **Do not fill your grocery cart with bad processed foods!!** I hear women all the time say they have to keep snacks for their children and then they eventually give in to eating the processed snacks themselves. Don't buy the processed snacks! Your children's developing bodies do not need that unhealthy garbage either! This is a great time for you to set a good example and also to teach your children how to make healthy snack choices. Recipes abound for making quick kid-friendly snacks from whole foods. Make your journey a family affair. Your family might not be thrilled to join, but it certainly won't damage them.

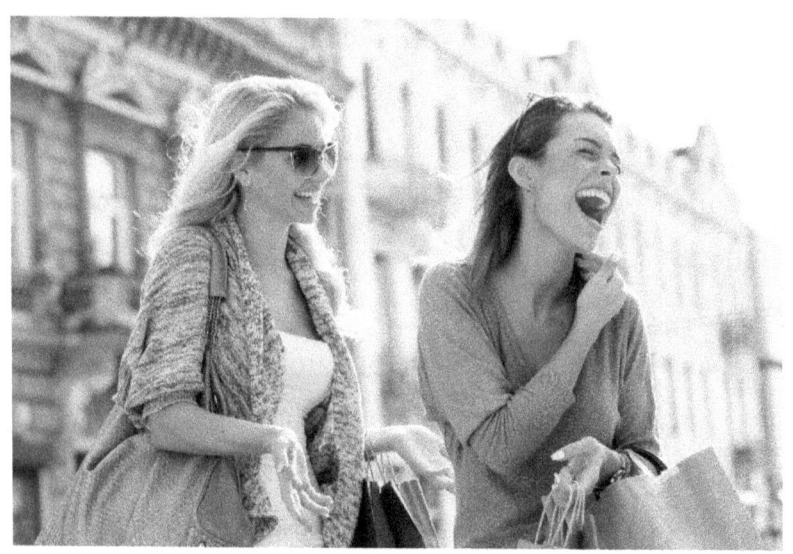

Honestly, we are all going to fail sometimes. That's part of life – it's part of learning. You are going to be making changes in many areas on your journey to better health, and it won't be healthy until you find the balance that makes you happy.

You won't always be perfect, but your efforts are going to make you stronger.

You'll be taking care of your physical and mental health, and you will be proud of the woman you find in the mirror.

Diet --- Ugh

The word "diet" conjures those negative thoughts, I know. <u>It's because diets don't work.</u> They come with rules and all sorts of unrealistic expectations that we can't follow long-term.

We naturally want to find a way to make them easy, to cheat. A healthy lifestyle means no need to cheat because you work to achieve a balance that you can maintain your whole life. Counting calories does not work because we automatically think we are being deprived.

If you make good dietary choices from real whole foods, you won't need to count calories. You'll feel satisfied more easily even though you'll be eating less.

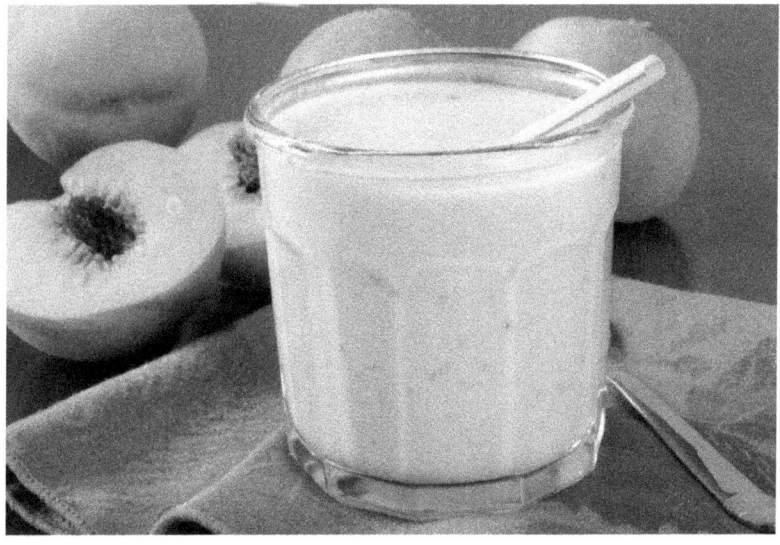

It can be overwhelming to consider a complete overhaul of our diet. Here is an adage that's helpful in getting started. It's from the late Dr. Annemarie Colbin who founded The Natural Gourmet Institute: "If it doesn't run, fly, swim, or grow from the ground, it's not food."

Don't worry about counting calories. Keep moderation in mind, but eat what you want of real food.

Stay away from items with a long list of ingredients and most certainly stay away from ingredients you can't identify.

Start being mindful about what you put in your body!

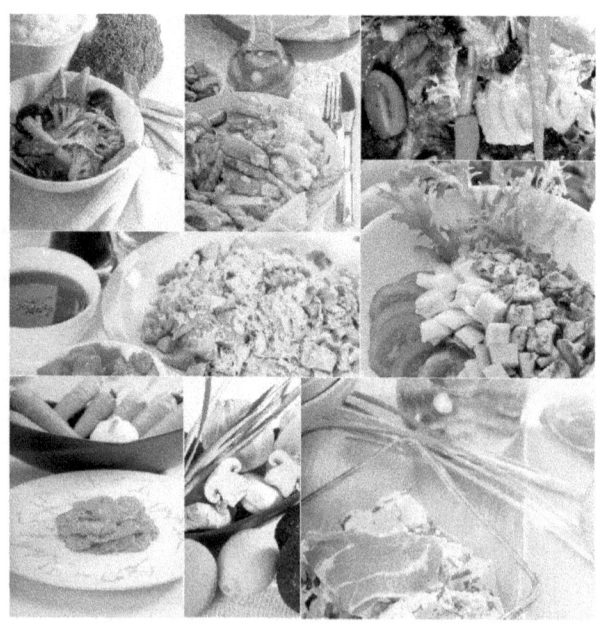

Build your meals around lean protein like chicken, turkey, seafood, eggs, nuts, venison, and lean beef (preferably grass fed) along with a variety of fruits and vegetables. Limit carbohydrates and eliminate processed food items and you'll experience amazing results quickly.

Another essential is preparing and cooking most of your meals at home. At home you are completely in control of what ingredients you use and how you cook.

When you do eat out, choose options that seem the least processed.

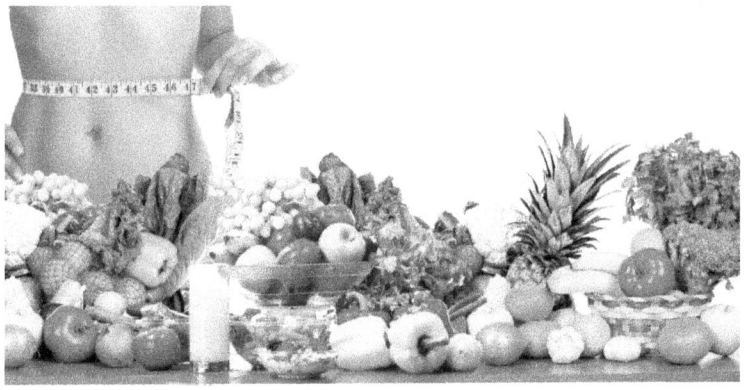

I would like to say there is a way to avoid the work and still be healthy, but alas I am afraid there is not.

A healthy, balanced life is going to mean you spend some time planning for what you will eat, shopping for it, and then cooking it at home.

I know, I know – we all work hard and we like for somebody to serve us and wait on us once in a while. This is a challenge for most of us, and it will really test your commitment on this journey to a healthier lifestyle.

Nothing wrong with a luncheon or night out to socialize and unwind, but as with every other part of life, we have to keep moderation in mind.

The majority of meals need to be prepared in your own kitchen. I promise you'll soon feel better and you'll be proud of your efforts!

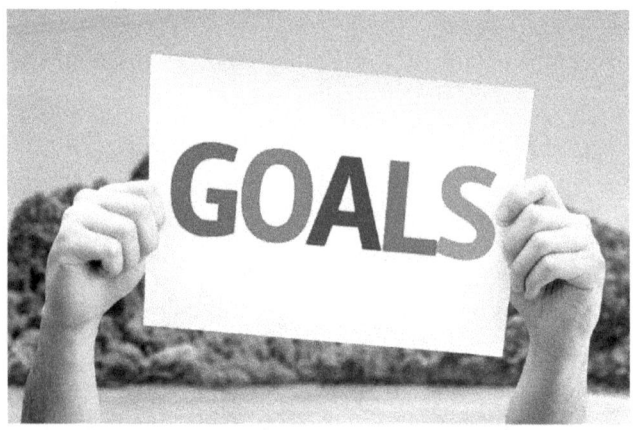

What this book offers you is not a prescribed diet, but some tips to acquire a healthier diet along with some suggestions that will help you avoid some of the pitfalls that might stymie your best results.

The first step to cleaning up your diet is cleaning out your kitchen! No matter how tempted you are to hoard those processed items that have a shelf-life of forever, don't do it.

If you can't stand the thought of them going to waste, donate them to a local food bank.

Let's consider some guidelines, tips, and suggestions for how to get rid of those items in your kitchen that are holding you back and leading to unhealthy habits.

1. Read labels! I'm warning you that you will be horrified at first when you realize what you've been putting in your body. Just because the packaging proclaims the item as healthy, does not mean it is. Many of the products well-known as "healthy" or "diet" are processed and preserved and contain high levels of sugar and salt --- and who knows what else. We can't even pronounce or identify most of what has been added to what might have once been something edible. They might be low in calories, but they are not beneficial to overall health. Stay away from items with genetically modified organism (GMO) ingredients. The jury is still out and the battle is still on about the effects of altering the genetic makeup of our food, but what is certain is nobody is sure what harm this stuff is really doing our bodies. It is a complex issue and it deserves your time. If you haven't read up on GMO's, you should do so and make decisions about what you are willing to accept in your diet. The best way to start eliminating these items is to look for "organic" or "non-GMO Project Verified" labels. Buy dairy and meats that are "grass fed" or "caught wild". Look for produce labeled

"vine ripened". Try it, and you'll be amazed how much better you feel.

2. Now, let's get the skinny on sugar: It's sweet goodness that we all need. The problem is we ingest way more than we need, and we typically have no idea how much or how often we put it in our bodies. The harmful effects of too much processed sugar would be another topic that really deserves your research. Being aware that it hides almost anywhere and realizing the negative effects of a sugary diet will be great motivation to clean it out. Here is an example for gauging your intake. The American Heart Association recommends women have 24 grams of sugar a day. About four teaspoons of sugar is equal to 1 gram. A brand name low-calorie/ low-fat container of yogurt has 18 grams of sugar. What you thought was a healthy snack, contains almost your entire daily recommended allowance of sugar. And, that soft drink you treated yourself with contains approximately 40 grams of sugar (some contain more). Now, who really has just one serving of a soft drink? They are bottled as 2 ½ servings. That's roughly 100 grams of sugar – WOW! Ever try munching on 25 teaspoons of sugar as a snack? – Bleh! Chances are if a product is labeled "low fat", sugar has replaced the fat and it isn't any healthier. Read labels and be aware of how much you are actually eating. We all need a little

sweetness in our lives, but too much is going to leave us feeling sick and unhappy. Go for healthier options like stevia, or munch on some fresh fruits. You can also use some honey or maple syrup. Occasional coconut or brown or cane sugar is also fine.

3. Stock your kitchen with fresh herbs and spices to replace salt. Even those of us who appear healthy can be damaging our bodies with too much salt. Guidelines recommend 1500 mg (3.75gm) – 2300 mg (6gm) of sodium a day for the average adult. Too much sodium has been proven to lead to heart disease, high blood pressure, stroke, kidney failure, and an assortment of other ailments. Salt is another ingredient that hides everywhere as a preservative. Those frozen "diet" entrées you pop in the microwave at lunch can have over 900 mg of sodium. Read labels to make sure you aren't ingesting your daily allowance in one meal. You'll find that seasoning food with a variety of other fresh herbs and spices will eliminate the need for salt as flavoring. If you retain water like most women do, salt will exacerbate the problem and make you appear bloated and heavier than you really are. Many women also report that they do not feel as hungry during the day once they reduce sodium intake. Many of us don't realize that the table salt we add to our food is actually processed and contains harmful chemicals. Look for

ways to eliminate or replace salt in your diet. Sea salt or Himalayan salt are better options because they are natural non-iodized and do have some health benefits ... when used in moderation.

4. If your goal is significant weight-loss, go gluten-free. Even if you don't experience full-blown allergic reactions to it, any sensitivity to it can hinder your weight-loss efforts. The truth is we all feel better without it, and it is in almost all processed foods. Plus, when you eliminate gluten, it forces you to choose whole foods in their natural form. Gluten is another item you need to educate yourself on so that you can make smarter choices in your diet. Research has proven that gluten-free / low- carb is the best diet for significant weight-loss. To learn more about gluten-free diets, I recommend you check out this blog where they offer a free eBook (healthy desserts, yum!) as a welcome gift:

www.kiraglutenfreerecipes.com

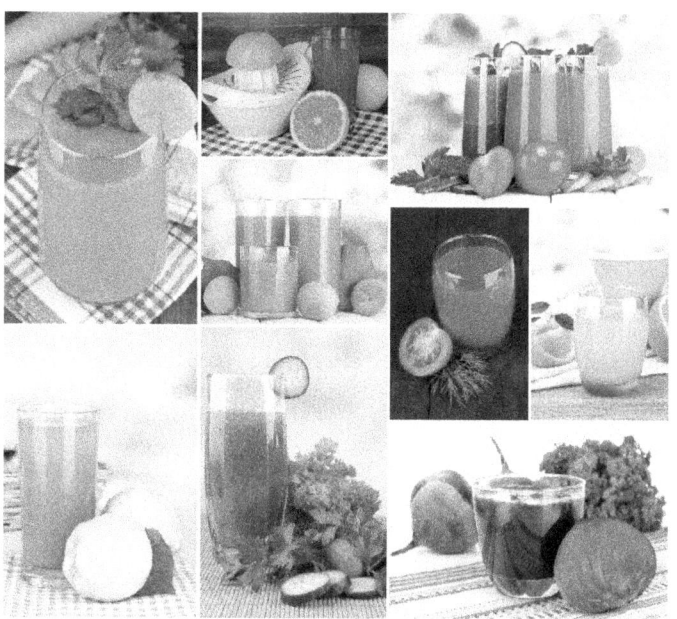

5. Stock up on superfoods and replace your less than healthy temptations with nutrient-rich foods that improve health and wellbeing. Some that have recently garnered superfood status are kale, spinach, broccoli, Brussel sprouts, blueberries, sweet potatoes, pomegranates, quinoa, salmon, almonds, ... Whew! Those are just a few to choose from. Kale (and most other leafy greens) provides more antioxidants than most other veggies, and along with broccoli and Brussel sprouts, it has detoxification powers that help your liver eliminate toxic by- products from your other not-so-healthy food choices. Kale is extra super because you

can eat it raw, saute it, broil it, steam it, or add it to a smoothie. Blueberries are also chock full off antioxidants, fiber, and Vitamin C. Pomegranates are also now being lauded for their cancer-fighting potential and proven ability to boost immunity. Sweet potatoes are rich in beta-carotene, potassium, and fiber, and are always considered a healthy tubular option. The Omega-3 fatty acids and amino acids in salmon boast a variety of health benefits that include decreased blood pressure and cholesterol, better vision, and repaired nerve damage. Winter squash is an excellent source of both beta-carotene and Omega-3's, along with the fiber that helps to fill you up. Chickpeas are another popular superfood. They are very low in fat and sodium, high in protein, iron, vitamins, fiber, and antioxidants. Mash them with some olive oil and herbs to make humus you enjoy with some broccoli or cauliflower for a super tasty and nutrient-rich snack! These are only a few superfood options, so you should definitely research and find some nutrient-rich foods you can add to your table. Enjoy these selections as a side or in a salad, soup, or smoothie. Think of it as using food as medicine. Don't cheat yourself! Start experiencing the benefits of these super powers in your diet! You can also recommend with powdered super foods such as chlorella, spirulina, or barley grass.

Alfalfa is also fantastic and it helps alkalize and detoxify the body.

6. Use only unsaturated or "good" fats. Not all fats are bad. Monounsaturated and polyunsaturated fats benefit heart health and insulin levels. They can make you feel full and curb cravings for "bad" fats that carry a variety of harmful effects for our bodies. Some good sources of unsaturated fats include unrefined olive oil and coconut oil, flaxseed oil, grapeseed oil, and nuts. Avocados and non-GMO tofu are other excellent choices of "good" fats. Almonds and walnuts are great sources of "good" fat and protein, so just a palm full can make you feel full and curb cravings. Try making condiments with these bases and flavored vinegars and lemon and lime juice. Remember moderation is the key to becoming healthier, so it is important to stay within the recommended daily allowance. The recommendation for women is that 20% - 35% of daily calories come from healthy sources of fat.

You are what you drink ... so, let's talk about that

None of us need an expert to tell us that the best drink is purified water and we should be drinking plenty of it. You don't have to look far to find the research supporting the detrimental effects of soft drinks and diet sodas.

Diet sodas are a chemical cocktail that should never be considered a healthy choice.

Fruit and vegetable juices can be processed with added sugar and sodium until the nutritional value is out the window.

As a matter of fact, you'll find your grocery store shelves full of choices claiming to be healthy drinks, but read the labels and you'll find an assortment of ingredients that are anything but. So, what do we drink?

Sometimes we need a little flavor and a little comfort from our daily liquid choices.

A good guideline is to think of drinks the way we think of food. Consider what nutritional value it offers.

1. Purified water is always the best choice. Adding some lemon or lime is adding some taste and nutritional value. Another healthy option is to fill the bottom of your glass with fresh fruits and add ice and water – healthy and refreshing. If you really enjoy fruit juice,

cut it in half with water for a lighter option that won't be so harsh on your body. Water is always our best drink choice and we need 6-8 8 ounce servings a day to reap all its benefits.

2. The subject of coffee is a murky one, indeed. One report will praise its super powers while another will warn of it catastrophic effects. Again, the key here is moderation. If it is a must in your life, one to two cups a day seems to be the recommendation in order to experience its benefits and none of its harm. Unfortunately, not only do we tend to drink too much of it, we tend to add a lot of sugary and fatty flavor to it that ends up making something natural another chemical cocktail we swallow down. Drinking it black, either hot or over ice, is best; but if you need flavor, try coconut or almond milk as creamer --- fewer calories and just as much flavor.

3. Tea is an excellent option that you can sip on throughout your day. A warm mug on chilly days can provide that same comfort you get from coffee, and green tea and chai tea are antioxidants packed with nutritional value. Sip some green tea hot or over ice and you'll feel energized and more alert. Its medicinal

value has also been linked to both heart disease and cancer prevention. Chai tea has been found to support digestion, prevent cancer, lower blood sugar and promote cardiovascular health. It also contains anti-inflammatory agents that give it medicinal properties as well. You are going to find your grocery shelves abounding with varieties of both these popular teas – every flavor imaginable has been concocted. Be sure to read labels and make certain you are buying natural forms. Just like with food choices, if you can't identify the ingredients, let it go.

4. Here's another murky topic: alcohol consumption. Clearly we all know the hazards of consuming too much – clearly the topic of another book - let's just look at it from the perspective of diet and feeling healthier. Research will say it makes you fat and research will say it can help you lose weight. It might cause cardiovascular problems or it might improve cardiovascular health. The issue is that it affects each of us differently, so the magic word again is "moderation." Moderation for women is considered one drink a day or no more than 6 – 8 drinks a week. If your goal is to lose weight, it's best to eliminate alcohol or make low calorie choices. Even if the alcohol we consume isn't adding pounds, it tends to lower our inhibitions, so we eat

more than we might normally consume. It also causes us to retain water that will hang around for days! If you want to drink moderately, continue to choose lower calorie options like lite beer, vodka with tonic water, or red wine which is proven to have a variety of health benefits when enjoyed in moderation. Avoid adding mixes and fruit juices that are full of sugar, sodium, and harmful chemicals.

More tips for natural weight loss drinks:

Start juicing vegetables and leafy greens. Invest in a quality juicer, like Omega Juicer.

Treat yourself to one nutritious vegetable juice a day. The best juicing recipes for weight loss include cucumbers, fennel, spinach, beets, tomatoes and ginger. You can season your juices with some Himalayan salt to taste. Keep hydrated and nicely energized!

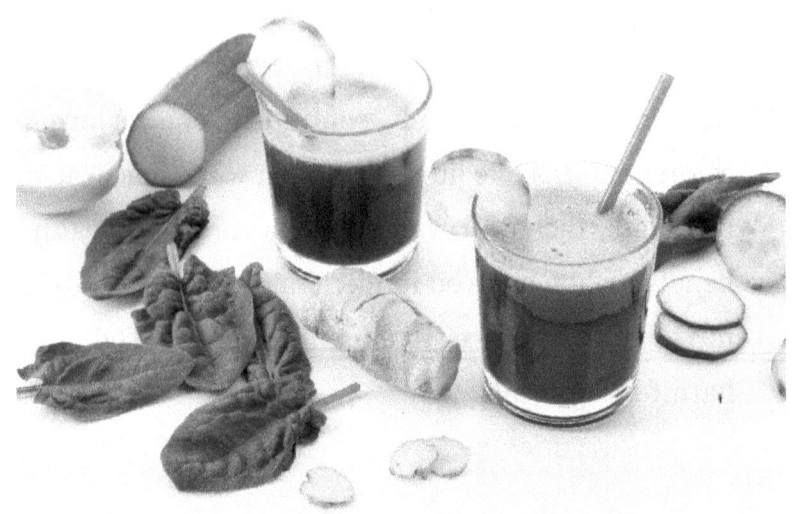

"The body is like a piano, and happiness is like music. It is needful to have the instrument in good order."

Henry Ward Beecher (1813 – 1887)

Ah, how to keep the body in good order when you are trying to keep everything else in good order? It's a challenge for sure, and this is where those of us with even the best intentions often give up on realizing our potential to be strong, healthy women.

This is also where that image of a tall, thin supermodel that we will never be squashes our efforts to be the best that we can be. Exercise shouldn't be about making you skinny; it should be about making you strong.

It should be about fine tuning you into the best instrument you can be. We let ourselves get discouraged by our failures to reach unrealistic expectations and we give up on the process that could be so beneficial to our overall health.

Exercise and physical activity are essential for a happy, healthy lifestyle.

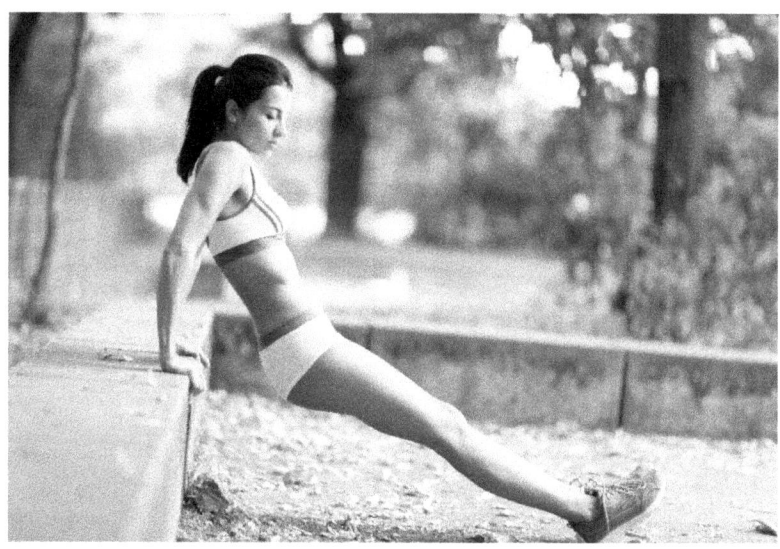

Consider these benefits to an active lifestyle: Exercise makes you happier – really, it does! Exercise is like a <u>free antidepressant</u>. It's been proven to reduce stress and anxiety, plus relieve depression and sleep deprivation. You'll have more energy during the day and sleep better at night. You'll be proud of even the small milestones that you reach, and that pride will make you more confident in other areas of your life. Research is revealing that regular exercise is also instrumental in preventing Alzheimer's and dementia.

It's not just important to our physical health, it's essential for maintaining our mental health as well.

If that isn't enough motivation, consider that it significantly improves your sex life. That's right. Regular exercise not only gives you more energy for a healthy sex life, it also improves your appearance and self-esteem making you feel more desirable.

A good workout triggers endorphins and adrenaline that boost your vitality, desire, and capacity for sexual activity. Get your partner on board for regular exercise and workout together. You'll enjoy double benefits!

> "My job is to be fit and I'm really blessed that I get to go and work out and live a really healthy lifestyle."- Kerri Walsh

Here's more motivation – regular exercise is a major part of taking care of yourself so that you can effectively and successfully perform all the other duties in your busy life. Our bodies are not meant for the sedentary lifestyle we have created.

The body is a huge muscle that needs to be constantly stretched and toned. The heart and lungs are muscles that will atrophy if we don't use them to their capacity.

You should do something every day that gets your heart rate up and causes you to breathe deeply. Don't wait for the day when you think it might come easily for you. That day won't come and you'll never realize how strong you really are.

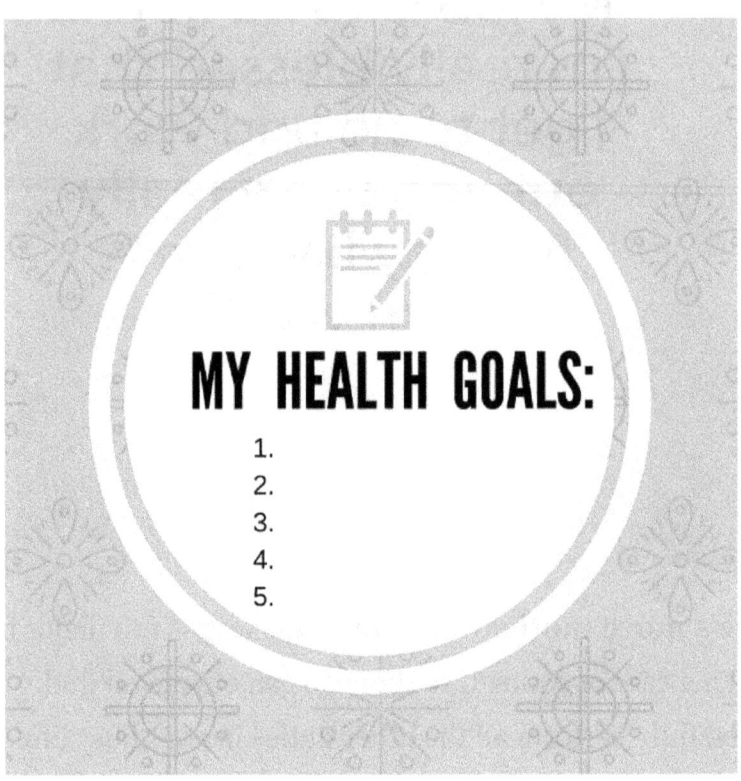

So, how do you get started leading a more active lifestyle? Just like you did with your diet, consider where you are right now and plan where you can make changes to include more physical activity in your day.

How many days a week do you exercise now? Are you leading a completely sedentary lifestyle? Are you active but need to add muscle tone to become stronger? Have you ever practiced a regular exercise program? Think about what motivated you to consider becoming more physically active. Do you want to look better? Feel better? Enjoy improved health? Now, make some short-term and long-term goals and let's get started! <u>You deserve to feel well and strong!</u>

No matter where you are on the fitness spectrum, you can add some physical activity that will help you lead a healthier life. Think about it like this – fit women are not in the gym working to get skinny and attractive; they are in the gym maintaining their healthy beautiful bodies.

There won't be a day when all your goals are met and you can quit exercising. You have to commit to it as an essential part of your overall healthier life.

It's extremely important that you find an activity you enjoy, so that daily exercise doesn't feel like another chore. Find an activity that produces beneficial emotional effects for you as well as physical. If you feel good about doing it, you'll be more likely to make it a habit.

If your lifestyle is currently pretty sedentary, ease into activities that you find enjoyable and increase duration and intensity as you become stronger.

Many of us self-sabotage right away because we try programs and routines that are too difficult for our current fitness level. We injure ourselves or our muscles are so sore we can't function for a few days, so once we recover we don't want to go back to whatever it was. You'll experience more long-term success if you ease into an exercise program that you enjoy.

The best routine for women to experience a real transformation in their bodies is a combination of cardio and weight training.

The American Heart Association recommends 30 minutes of cardiovascular activity a day. The Center for Disease Control recommends 150 minutes a week. Now, if you aren't ready for 30 minutes, do what you can!

If you are beginning and you need to start with 15 minutes, you'll soon find yourself capable of 30 minutes and more. You'll be building a habit that will render great rewards.

Carving time for Cardio

Most of us lead such busy lives we really don't have time for a gym membership or a personal trainer. And, let's be honest, if you are out of shape or not feeling confident about your skill level, gyms are intimidating.

So, how do we fit in 30 minutes to an hour for cardio in every day? Walking, jogging, biking, gardening, swimming, and dancing are all great aerobic activities that can be done with family and friends. If you are having trouble getting started, consider your daily activities and find where one of these would naturally fit.

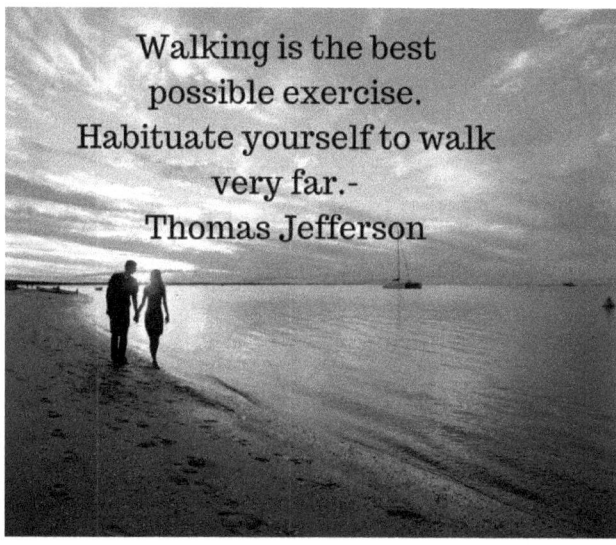

Some of us have to make the commitment to rising 30 minutes earlier and getting it in before we start our day. If that's not an option, think about times in your day when you are sedentary and consider how you could fill those minutes with exercise.

Taking the baby or your dog for a walk or jog in the afternoon would have great benefits for all. If you are shuttling kids to sports practices, take a 30 -minute walk or jog while you wait.

Most practices are an hour, so you'll still have time to watch Jr. kick the soccer ball around, and you might find other moms joining you. It won't take long and you'll be walking a little longer, a little farther, and a little faster.

If you watch television in the evening, don't be a couch potato! Find ways to break a sweat while you catch up on *Grey's Anatomy!*

They have televisions in gyms for a reason; working out can be boring and watching is a good distraction.

You will probably find that you exercise longer because you are engrossed in whatever show you are watching.

Keep your workout equipment near the television and pull it out while you watch. Use dumbbells, resistance bands, or a medicine ball and strength train.

Or, jog in place, do crunches, jumping jacks, leg lifts, toe touches, or lunges. Break a sweat!

Another good activity to get started is dancing. Can't make it to a Zumba class? Turn on your favorite playlist and dance around the house while you complete some of your evening chores.

You don't see many dancers who aren't in shape because it's difficult and it burns calories. Fit Radio is a popular free app that provides playlists in a variety of genres geared toward exercise.

Buying a premium package allows you to make your own lists, but the free lists are great for beginners.

Challenge yourself to dance through a whole list or a certain number of songs. Pretty soon you'll be ready for a more challenging activity.

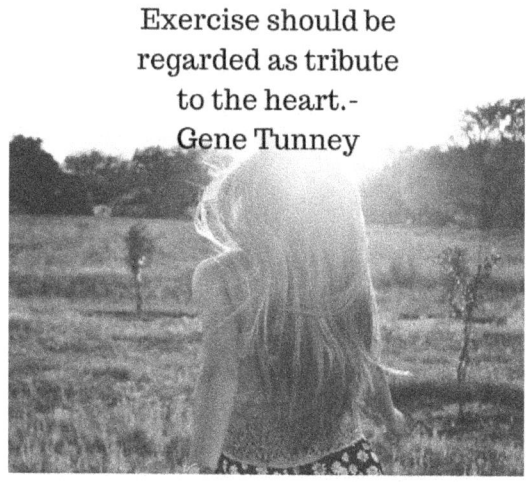

Exercise should be regarded as tribute to the heart. - Gene Tunney

Here's another idea – turn on your computer! YouTube abounds with workout videos for everybody.

You can find the 4-minute, 7-minute, and 10- minute workout sequence for almost any activity at any skill level. Full workouts for strength training and full-body cardio are right at your fingertips. Of course, you'll want to research and make sure they are produced by experts, but plenty feature popular renowned fitness experts with years of experience. It's like having a professional trainer in your home at your convenience.

And, as we mentioned earlier, if it exists, there's an app for it. Many of the fitness apps available allow you to choose the type of exercise you need and then customize your routine ...

FOR FREE! Use the technology you have available to help you get started moving during the day.

Building Muscle

For decades we've been skipping out on weight training by using the excuse that we don't want to bulk up and look manly. So, we've been missing out on the benefits of a toned body with lean muscle mass.

Women don't typically have the hormones required to pack on bulky muscle, so unless you are planning to take supplements and train like a bodybuilder, you needn't worry about a few hours a week lifting light weights turning you into The Hulk.

Plus, we all have to admit we envy those women who are a little bit older and are still looking good in tanks and sleeveless blouses. We'd all like to look more toned and confident.

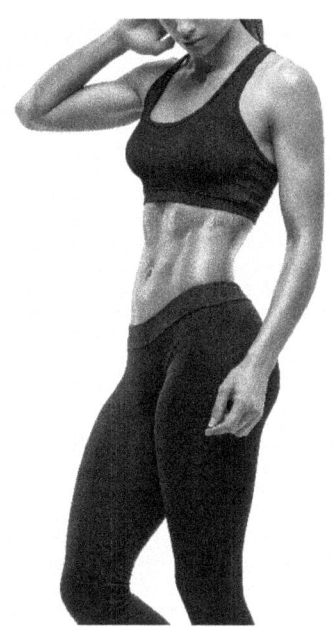

If you really want to transform your body and get stronger, you'll have to hit the weights. It's recommended for women to strength train for 20-30 minutes 2-3 days a week.

However, whatever time you can get in is going to be very beneficial to your overall health and appearance, and you do not need a gym membership to get started. Toned muscle burns fat and calories.

You'll burn more calories and your body will look leaner than it will if you stick to just cardio workouts. Also, a little strength training helps us maintain our posture and fight Osteoporosis.

The good news is we can build muscle as long as we live, so it's never too late to start.

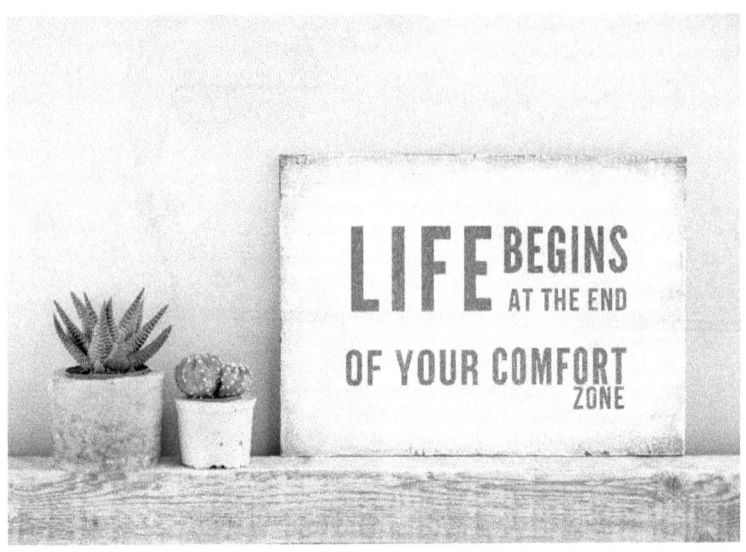

Start with weights light enough that you can complete sets of 12-15 repetitions. It won't take long before you'll be ready to move to heavier weights and try adding new moves. Dumbbells are perfect for getting started, but resistance bands, medicine balls, or kettle balls are great choices too.

These often come with instructions for suggested exercises and routines. If you aren't ready for any of those, do the recommended reps using soup cans.

If you follow through, you'll be surprised at how quickly you will feel confident enough to increase the weight. I promise – you'll see results and you'll like what you see.

Exercising Your Soul

If there is anything we women fail to take care of more than our bodies, it's our minds. Our day is filled with rushing from place to place, solving problems at home and at work, caring for others, and then dealing with our own burdens and emotional baggage.

Who can keep up with it all? We lie down at night with our mind still spinning with the problems of the day, so then we don't sleep well.

We wake up still physically and emotionally fatigued and ill-equipped to deal with the next day's drama – another vicious circle that becomes our life.

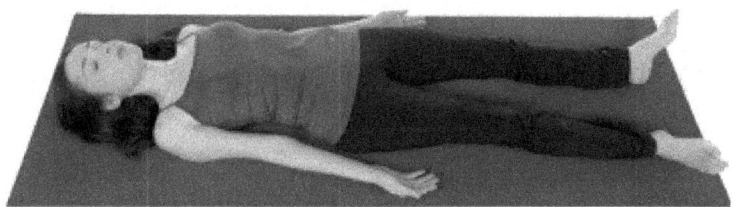

As important as it is to clean the toxins from our bodies, it's even more important to clean them from our mind.

The good news is it really only takes minutes to let go of negative thoughts and clear the junk from your head.

Practicing just a few minutes of some type of quiet time or meditation will decrease stress and anxiety, help you sleep, and increase your spiritual connection.

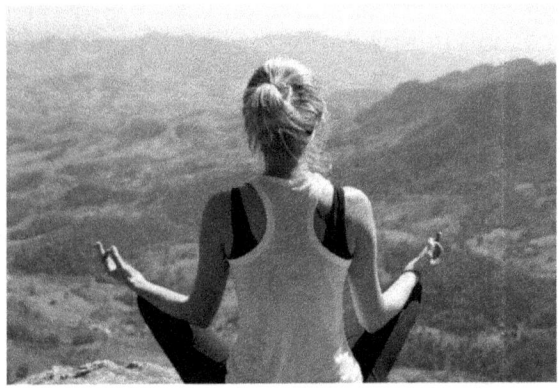

The problem is we don't like silence. We are afraid of silence, so we strive to fill up every second of our lives with noise.

We often express the need for quiet, but when given the chance we don't take it. We seek out noise to fill the emptiness. Taking just a few minutes to silence your mind gives it a chance to renew and create order out of the chaos of the day.

It's a way to nourish your soul, and taking time to do it will make you so much more productive in every part of your life. It takes practice and it takes commitment.

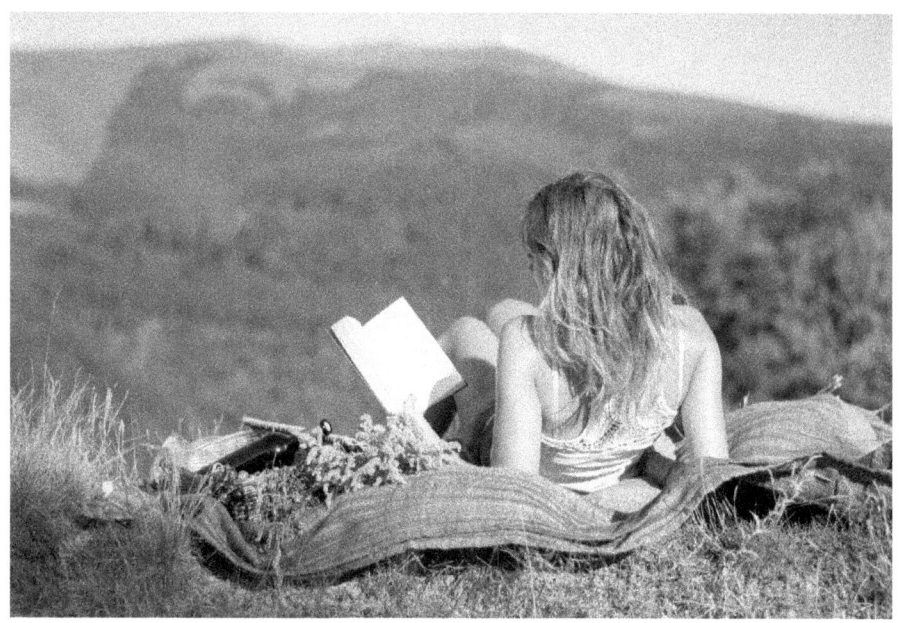

Society is so fast paced and we are so bombarded by constant images and noises, it's hard to find the time and place to be alone and refresh.

If you feel your life is too hectic to find quiet, start by committing just 2-3 minutes a day. Once you experience the amazing effects of what you find in quiet, you'll begin making more time to renew your mind and spirit.

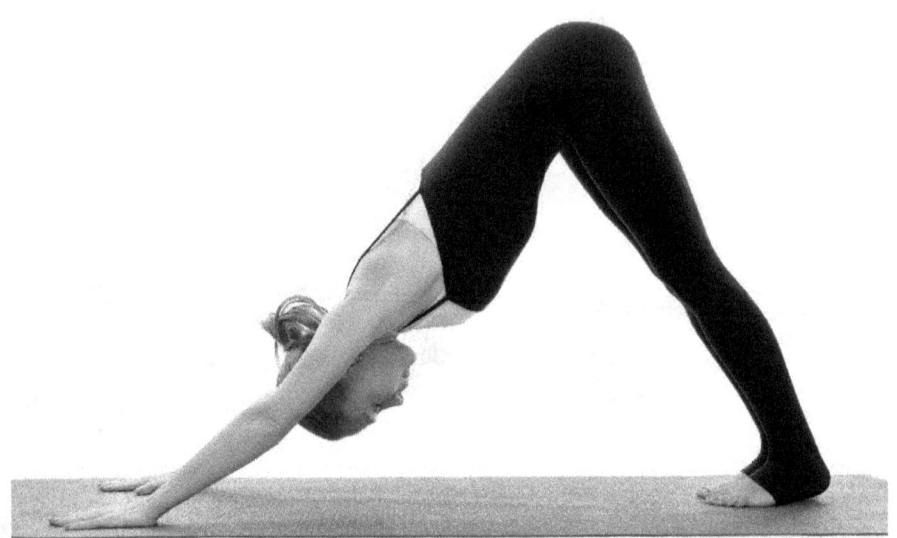

It can also be a little naturally overwhelming to commit to doing nothing, but it's so important for our body and soul.

It's a prescribed therapy for those who seek mental health counseling because it allows us to center and really find ourselves when we get lost in the chaos of life.

Some planning before you get started can ensure it's an enjoyable and successful experience.

1. Plan a place – I know, easier said than done. But, it can be done. Think of somewhere you are most comfortable that is accessible every day – somewhere free from distraction. Many women immediately choose the bathtub – nothing like a warm bath! Other suggestions

are a place outdoors, a sauna, your favorite chair, wherever you feel relaxed.

2. Schedule a time. You'll be more likely to commit if you view it as an appointment. If you only have 2-3 minutes to spare for silent breathing, start there. Anytime you give yourself to slow down and center will be helpful to your overall wellbeing.

3. Decide what you hope to accomplish from the time you spend. Do you need to calm yourself down after a hectic day? Do you want a stronger spiritual connection? Do you need relaxation for better sleep? Do you need a better sense of self? Thinking about what your needs are can help you plan a method for meditation.

4. Here's the most important: Decide how you want to spend this time. If you have no idea where to start, practice deep breathing. Maybe you need to spend it in prayer. Many people find peace in repeating a positive phrase in their head like a mantra while forcing all other thoughts out. Yoga is a wonderful practice that exercises the body and soul. If you've never tried it, you should. Do some research and you'll find plenty of beginner sessions online. It can be practiced without

any equipment and effective sessions can only take minutes. It's a beautiful practice that makes you feel strong and confident.

However you choose to spend this time, make sure you are as disciplined about it as you are exercising your body. Don't feel guilty about taking a few minutes to renew your mind. It is just as important to your health and it's an integral part of taking care of ourselves.

Sleep, Where Art Thou?

Six to eight hours of sleep a night is recommended for women. We all know that very few of us get enough sleep to be healthy and productive.

We all have our personal demons that haunt us at night and keep sleep at bay.

However, most women discover that once they take the time to take care for themselves and begin balancing their lives, sleeping patterns are greatly improved.

To be honest, we all know that sleep issues are very complex and can be multifactorial. Some issues that deprive us of sleep are hormone related and some stem from diagnosed medical problems.

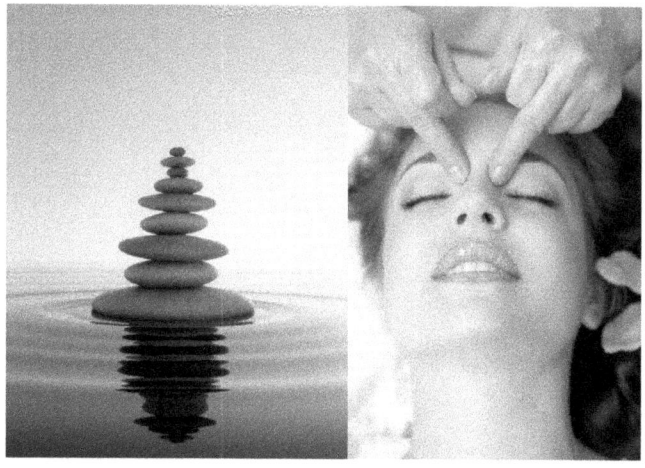

But, some can be regulated with lifestyle changes. Exercising to tire your body and then practicing deep breathing to relax it can be very effective.

Once you begin living a lifestyle filled with healthy food, daily exercise and activity, and meditation, you'll be amazed at how easily sleep will come.

Proper sleep and rest are so important for a happy, fulfilled life. Take care of yourself and make sure you give yourself enough sleep.

If you feel you need help, seek it! It's part of taking control of your own wellbeing.

Sign Up for Our Email Newsletter and Get a Free eBook

www.yourwellnessbooks.com/newsletter

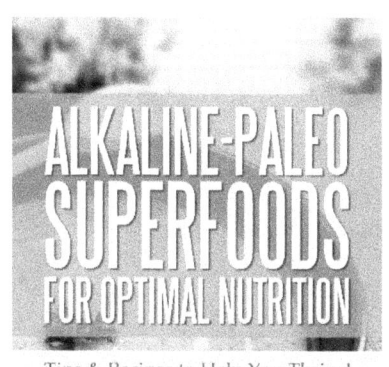

Closing

The journey toward a better self is a life journey. Once these new choices become habits, it'll be an easy road to follow. You'll feel so good about yourself and you'll want to continue experiencing all the benefits of a balanced, healthy life.

Don't think of these practices as a means-to-an-end. They should become habits in your life that lead to a new more enjoyable lifestyle.

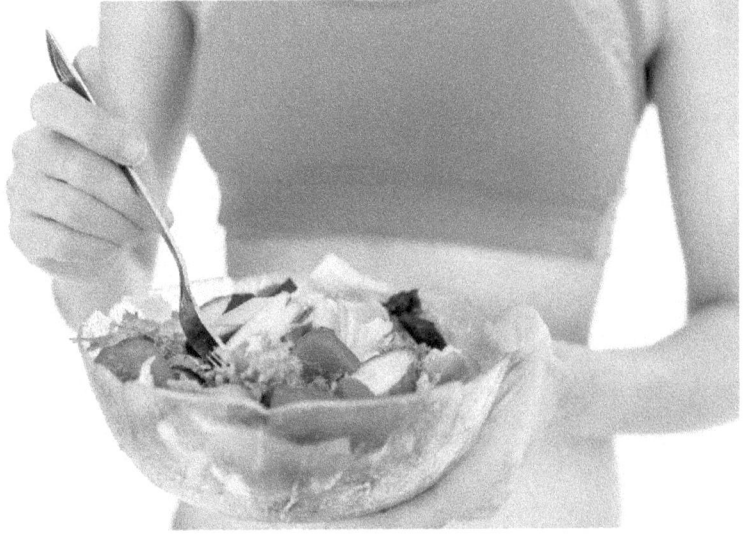

Decide today that you want to discover just how awesome you can be! Take the suggestions here that will help you and begin taking care of your physical, mental, and spiritual health. Love yourself and take responsibility for your own wellbeing. You deserve to be happy, fit, and strong!

To your success + enjoy the process!

Elena Garcia

Before I go, I need to ask you a favor. If you received any value from this book, could you please post an honest review and share with your friends?

I am always very excited to hear from my readers and your review can inspire other women to change their lifestyles, to get health and energy they deserve.

Thank You!

You can also reach me via email at:

elenajamesbooks@gmail.com

More Books by Elena Garcia (Kindle & Paperback)

Available at:

www.YourWellnessBooks.com

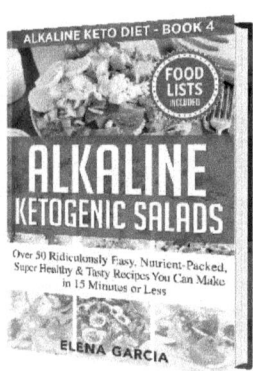
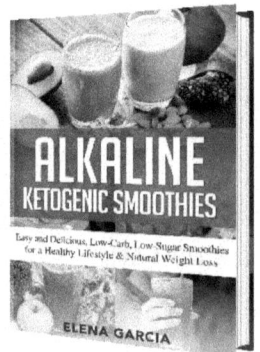
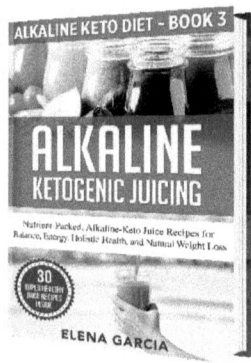
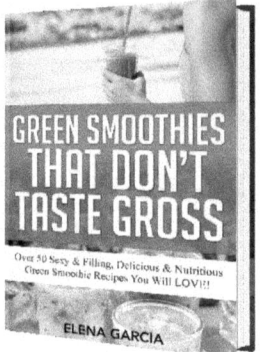

www.ingramcontent.com/pod-product-compliance
Lightning Source LLC
Chambersburg PA
CBHW071126030426
42336CB00013BA/2212